$50 SAVED
MY LIFE

$50 SAVED MY LIFE

MALA BALRAM SLOWE

Library of Congress Control Number: 2024907679

ISBN: 979-8-89228-121-8   (Paperback)
ISBN: 979-8-89228-122-5   (eBook)

Book Ordering Information:
Atticus Publishing
548 Market St PMB 70756
San Francisco, CA 94104
(888) 208-9296
info@atticuspublishing.com
www.atticuspublishing.com

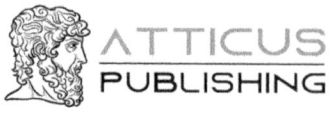

Printed in the United States of America

Contents

PART 1

Parties and Priorities

CHAPTER 1

The Wellness Check

It was Friday, Labor Day weekend in 2018, and I was finishing work as a medical coordinator at the hospital. My coworker Mary approached me with an intriguing question.

"Hey, did you get your $50.00?" Mary asked with a mischievous smile.

I was taken aback. "Wait, $50.00? What are you talking about?" I inquired, my curiosity piqued.

Just as I was about to delve into the details, the ringing of my phone interrupted the conversation. I hastily picked it up, balancing the receiver between my shoulder and ear, and my daughter, Stephanie's, voice filled my ears.

"Hey, Mom, are you available for dinner tonight?" Stephanie asked eagerly. I considered my plans for the evening. "Well, I have a few other places to go, but let's do dinner first. I'll make time for you," I replied warmly before ending the call.

With the phone call behind me, I turned back to Mary. My curiosity about the $50.00 rekindled. As if reading my mind, she explained that the insurance we had taken out provided a wellness benefit. If we underwent a wellness check, we would receive $50.00 as a reward.

The idea of receiving some extra cash immediately sparked my interest, and I expressed my eagerness to participate; my eyes widened with excitement. "That sounds amazing! I want to get that wellness check and claim that

$50.00," I exclaimed.

However, my excitement was quickly replaced with disappointment as I realized I had already completed all the wellness checks for the year. Disheartened, I sighed, thinking that I had missed out on the opportunity to earn some extra cash.

But Mary, ever resourceful, had a solution. "There's one test you haven't done yet," she revealed, a glimmer of hope in her eyes.

Curiosity once again ignited within me. "Which test am I missing?" I asked apprehensively.

Mary looked at me earnestly and suggested, "You should go get a mammogram done. It's recommended when you turn forty, and it's part of our insurance wellness benefits."

I hesitated, convinced that I had no symptoms or pain and thus saw no need for a mammogram. I balked at the suggestion, confidently asserting, "No, I'm fine. I don't have any aches or pain."

However, the allure of the $50.00 lingered in my mind. As I sat at my desk, pondering over the potential reward, a thought crossed my mind. Despite my initial reluctance, I reasoned, "Well, it's Friday before Labor Day," I mused. "I can use my lunch break and go get it done."

Determined to seize the opportunity, I made my way to the nearby breast center. Nervous but hopeful, I underwent the mammogram, the prospect of the $50.00 incentive driving me forward. When it was over, I felt a sense of relief and happiness. I knew I had taken a proactive step toward my well- being.

Returning to the office, I filled out the necessary paperwork and submitted it, a smile of satisfaction adorning my face. I turned to Mary and expressed my gratitude, saying, "I'm glad you told me to go get this done. I wanted that

$50.00, but more importantly, I feel accomplished."

As the day came to a close, I received a call signaling the end of my shift. I informed Mary of my plans for the evening. "Well, I'm heading out to lots of parties this weekend, but first, I'm having dinner with Stephanie," I shared with a hint of excitement in my voice.

Over the weekend, my social calendar brimmed with invitations from friends and family, promising a whirlwind of excitement and memorable experiences. The festivities began on Friday night with a lively birthday celebration that extended into the early hours of Saturday morning. The atmosphere was electric, filled with laughter, music, and the joy of celebrating another year of a dear friend's life. As the clock struck 2:30 a.m., I bid farewell to the party, my heart still buzzing with the infectious energy of the night.

But the weekend had only just begun, and there was another event on the horizon that had everyone buzzing with anticipation. Raj, a close friend known for throwing legendary parties, was hosting an extravaganza that promised an unforgettable experience. The mere mention of Raj's party set pulses racing and filled the air with excitement.

Eager to make the most of the weekend, I picked up the phone and called my friends, organizing the details and ensuring that we would be ready for the evening's festivities. The plan was set: I would swing by and pick them up at 8:00 p.m. The anticipation grew as we shared our excitement and prepared for a night of revelry and celebration.

As I embarked on a weekend filled with festivities and cherished moments, little did I know that my decision to undergo that mammogram would have a far greater impact on my life than I could have ever imagined.

CHAPTER 2

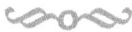

Nurturing Bonds

As the night progressed, I sat down for dinner with my daughter, Stephanie over our meal, Stephanie brought up the topic of Thanksgiving, expressing her desire for me and Jerry, my boyfriend, to visit her at her new apartment.

"When are you going to come visit me at my new place?" Stephanie asked, her eyes filled with anticipation. "I want you and Jerry to come over for Thanksgiving dinner this year." She hoped we would join her for Thanksgiving dinner, envisioning a warm family gathering.

I asked Stephanie who would be cooking the Thanksgiving dinner at her new place, and she replied with excitement, "Dad is going to cook for us!"

My heart sank as I listened to her response. A wave of conflicting emotions washed over me, and I hesitated before gathering the courage to speak my truth. "Actually," I said, hesitating for a moment, unsure how to respond, "well, actually, I was planning on going to Auntie's house for Thanksgiving," I finally admitted.

It was as if a storm cloud had suddenly descended upon our conversation, casting a shadow over the moment. She tried to mask her emotions. Stephanie nodded understandingly, though a hint of disappointment flickered across her face.

"I see," she said softly, her voice tinged with sadness. "So you don't want to have dinner with us then?"

My heart ached at her words, knowing that they held a deeper meaning. The realization of the impact my decision had on my daughter hit me like a ton of bricks. In that moment, I understood the weight of my choice and the hurt it caused her.

I took a deep breath, trying to steady myself as I met her gaze. Feeling a pang of guilt, I quickly reassured her, my voice filled with remorse, "It's not that, sweetheart. I just had already made plans. But I promise we'll find another time to have a special meal together."

Tears welled up in Stephanie's eyes as she searched my face, looking for sincerity in my words. A surge of emotion washed over me, and I reached out to hold her hand, squeezing it gently. A faint smile graced her lips. In that moment, it felt as if a heavy burden had been lifted, and a flicker of hope ignited within me.

Curiosity sparked within me, and I asked Stephanie about her weekend plans. She mentioned going shopping and hanging out with friends, a typical routine for a young woman enjoying her independence. In turn, she questioned my own plans.

"What are you doing this weekend, Mom?" she inquired.

"I'm going to pick up my friends and go over to Sean's and Raj's house tonight," I replied, a hint of excitement in my voice. "Then tomorrow during the day, I'm going Labor Day shopping and having lunch with Jerry. And in the evening, we're going to a club. Oh, and don't forget that

Monday is your cousin Jay's birthday party. You mustn't miss it!"

Stephanie's eyes widened as she absorbed my packed schedule. Concern laced her voice as she said, "Mom, you're always so busy, going out and about. How do you have so many friends and social engagements?"

I smiled, understanding her perspective. "Well, my dear, I have a lot of friends and a free-spirited nature. I love life and embrace every moment. Plus, I'm grateful that Jerry treats me like a queen. I have a fulfilling job, wonderful friends, and a loving family. What more can one ask for?"

But Stephanie has been pointing out how busy I always seemed to be. She gently expressed her feelings and voiced her desire for more quality time together. She pointed out how my calendar seemed filled to the brim with social events and family gatherings. She felt a pang of resentment, feeling that I prioritized socializing over quality mother-daughter bonding. She yearned for undivided attention.

Her words struck a chord deep within me, and I swallowed hard, realizing the truth in her words. I acknowledged her feelings and promised to make an effort to have a dedicated mother-daughter day at least once a month. "I'm sorry if you feel this way, Stephanie. I do have a lot of commitments, but I understand now how important it is to have dedicated mother-daughter days. I promise I will make it a priority from now on." Her request resonated within me, reminding me of the importance of nurturing our relationship amid the busyness of life.

Our conversation took an unexpected turn, as Stephanie shifted gears, asking about her Christmas gift, already making her wishes known. She had her eye on a new MacBook and hoped I would save up to buy it for her. I listened attentively, acknowledging her request without making any immediate promises. I reminded her that she had received a MacBook just a year ago, but she insisted she needed a new one. She then shared her plans to go to Disney for Christmas with her father. "Daddy and I are planning to go to Disney for Christmas, so it would be great if I could have my gift before then."

Her request was met with a chuckle, though I could sense her genuine anticipation. "Well, sweetheart, I can't promise anything just yet," I responded with a playful tone. "But let's see how things go. Remember, it's the thought that counts."

Stephanie's laughter echoed, and for a moment, I felt a wave of relief wash over me. It was a reminder that amid the chaos of our lives, we could still find joy and laughter in the simplest of conversations.

As the conversation wound down, I assured her. "I'll consider it, Stephanie," I replied, trying to strike a balance between fulfilling her wishes and managing expectations and promised to work on spending more time together.

I worked to repair the rift that had unintentionally formed between Stephanie and me. We sat down together, engaging in heartfelt conversations, and slowly began to heal the wounds caused by misunderstandings and diverging paths.

Wanting to delve deeper into her life, I inquired about her work, and she admitted her discontent with her job. We continued our conversation until the waiter arrived with the bill, and I reassured Stephanie, "I've got this covered, and we will work on spending more time together. I love you."

With a mix of emotions and a newfound determination, I left the restaurant that evening. I knew that nurturing our bond and prioritizing my role as a mother were essential steps toward finding the balance between my social life and my responsibilities.

It was time to show Stephanie that she was truly cherished and loved. I realized the importance of forgiveness, understanding, and the resilience of family. We cherished the love that had brought us together, and creating new memories that would forever shape our journey forward.

CHAPTER 3

Sean's Sensational Soiree

The phone rang, and Ann's voice filled the air with excitement, "Where are you guys? Are you ready? I'll be there in twenty minutes!"

Anticipating a night of celebration, Jasmine and Ann quickly hopped into the car. As they drove, Ann and Jasmine engaged in lively conversation, discussing which party they should attend first.

"I think we should go to Sean's party first and then head over to Jay's," Jasmine suggested, sharing the details she had heard. "Jay's party is supposed to go on until 6:00 a.m., and they're even having a live band!"

The pulsating sound of music greeted us as we arrived at Sean's party. The energy was infectious, and I couldn't resist surrendering to its rhythm. Excitement buzzed through the crowd as I greeted familiar faces and made new acquaintances.

"Hey, Sean! How's it going?" Jasmine exclaimed, fully embracing the party atmosphere. The place was packed with unfamiliar faces too, leaving me curious.

"I wonder where Sean met all these people," I asked Ann.

"I'm not a fan of this music," Ann murmured to Jasmine, her disappointment evident. "I don't think we'll be staying here for long."

Jasmine, always up for a good time, suggested they grab a drink. "Let's have a drink and see how it goes," she proposed, her eyes gleaming mischievously. "I'll take a double vodka with a splash of soda."

Amused by Jasmine's request, Ann chimed in, "Why do you even bother asking for soda? Just go all out!"

As the night progressed, the music intensified, and bodies moved in sync with the beat. Lost in the moment, I found myself dancing with newfound friends, reveling in the freedom of the night. Laughter and cheers filled the space, amplifying the sense of joy and camaraderie.

Jasmine, eager to let loose and dance, exclaimed, "Hey, I ran into an old friend! Let's have another drink, girls!"

Making my way to the bar, I ordered a drink and caught sight of Scott, a friend of Sean's whom I hadn't seen in years. Excited to reconnect, I joined him, reminiscing about old times and toasting to the night ahead.

As we ventured through the party, the drinks kept flowing, adding to the electrifying atmosphere. The night began to blur into a hazy whirlwind of music, laughter, and the company of friends.

Ann jokingly remarked, "I might get drunk before we even reach the next party!"

Jasmine, ever the party enthusiast, replied, "Well, it's going to be a long night. Let's make the most of it!"

Amid the revelry, hunger struck, and Jasmine suggested we take a break to eat. Arriving at the food spread, we marveled at the delicious offerings.

"Wow, this food looks amazing. Who cooked all this?" Jasmine inquired. "That's Sean's friend's mom," someone nearby replied. "They sure know how to throw an all-American feast!"

As they indulged in mouthwatering delicacies, Jasmine teased Ann about her anticipated lack of appetite. "Come on, Ann, you know you won't eat much. You need to have something to soak up the alcohol!"

Amused, Ann rolled her eyes and playfully responded, "All right, I'll make an effort, just for you!"

Amid the pulsating lights and contagious energy, I glanced over at Ann who seemed equally captivated by the party's allure. She beckoned me to join her for another drink, and together we ventured deeper into the crowd, embracing the euphoria of the moment.

The night carried on, filled with dancing, laughter, and the rhythmic beats of the music. They lost themselves in the moment, fully embracing the vibrant energy surrounding them. It felt like the party would never end.

However, as the music shifted and the night grew late, Ann's enthusiasm waned, and she expressed her dissatisfaction with the playlist. Eventually, exhaustion began to creep in, and Ann confessed, "I've had enough. It's time to go home."

Sensing her disinterest, we agreed it was time to move on to the next celebration. With a mixture of emotions and memories that would linger, we bid farewell to the party and made our way to the next event, eagerly anticipating what the night had in store.

CHAPTER 4

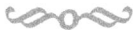

Jay's Unforgettable Bash

Leaving Sean's party behind, we embarked on a thrilling journey filled with raucous laughter and bubbling anticipation as we made our way to Jay's house. The car ride buzzed with electric excitement. The air crackling with the promise of an unforgettable night that seemed to pulsate through our veins.

Ann couldn't contain her enthusiasm as she dialed Jay's number. Her voice brimming with unbridled excitement. "I'm on my way to your house!" she exclaimed. Her words practically dancing with joy.

Jay's voice crackled through the phone, equally filled with anticipation. "Okay, I'm here with Deven," he replied. His voice laced with enthusiasm.

"We're on our way too. The more the merrier!" the anticipation in Ann's voice grew even stronger.

Arriving at Jay's house, we were immediately greeted by an explosion of vibrant sounds that enveloped the entire neighborhood. The music acted as a siren's call, drawing party-goers from far and wide, their curiosity piqued by the infectious energy that emanated from within. Parking proved to be an exhilarating challenge, but the pulsating energy of the night compelled us to find a way. Determination ignited, I turned to Jay, hoping for a solution.

"Hey, Jay, can I park on your grass?" I asked with a hint of desperation.

Jay's response was gracious and accommodating, a true reflection of his generous spirit. "Sure, go ahead," he replied with a warm smile, allowing me to park on his grass and ensuring that we wouldn't miss a single minute of the revelry.

Stepping inside Jay's house, we were immediately swept away by a whirlwind of excitement, finding ourselves submerged in a sea of jubilant revelers. Each person was fully immersed in the infectious rhythm and electric atmosphere that characterized the celebration. Jay's humble abode had undergone a remarkable transformation, becoming a haven of pulsating music, contagious laughter, and vibrant conversation. The tantalizing aroma of mouthwatering food permeated the air, teasing our taste buds and tempting us to indulge in the delectable spread.

As I surveyed the scene, I marveled at the stark contrast between Sean's party and Jay's gathering. Here, in this magical space, cultures merged and collided, creating a tapestry of celebration that was truly extraordinary. Indian cuisine adorned the tables, presenting a stunning fusion of traditional and contemporary flavors. We reveled in the sheer joy of embracing diverse culinary experiences, savoring each mouthwatering bite with deep appreciation.

"Let's raise a glass to the freaking weekend!" I enthusiastically exclaimed, seizing a drink in my hand. The music swirled and soared, filling the air with its intoxicating melodies, beckoning us to surrender ourselves to the rhythm and let loose. This was a party unlike any other, where the thumping bass and infectious beats ignited an irresistible urge to move our bodies and surrender to the vivacious energy that surrounded us. With each heartbeat aligning with the pulsating music, our souls became entwined in a symphony of euphoria.

As the night wore on, the music reached a crescendo, captivating our senses and casting a spell over the crowd. We danced with wild abandon, laughing uproariously, and embracing the spirit of unity that transcended cultural boundaries. It was a glorious testament to the profound power of shared experiences, reminding us of the resplendent beauty found in embracing diversity and forging connections that spanned continents and lifetimes.

The hours flew by, but it felt as if time had been suspended, elongating the fleeting moments of bliss. As we reveled in the festivities, we found ourselves immersed in the company of both friends and strangers. Their stories interwoven with ours, creating a tapestry of unforgettable memories. We laughed until tears streamed down our faces, sang along to every word, and danced with complete abandon. The night seemed infinite, a whirlwind of unadulterated joy, and uninhibited celebration.

As the first rays of dawn painted the sky in hues of pink and gold, signaling the end of the night's revelry, a bittersweet mix of exhaustion and contentment settled upon us. We couldn't help but carry a sense of profound fulfillment within our weary bones. Jay's unforgettable bash had surpassed our wildest expectations, leaving an indelible mark upon our hearts. It was a testament to the magic that unfurls when diverse worlds collide in harmonious celebration.

Reluctantly, we bid farewell to Jay's house, carrying with us the spirit of the night and the memories we had crafted. Our footsteps echoed with echoes of laughter, our hearts filled to the brim with the joys of the night. It was a party that would forever be etched in the deepest recesses of our souls, a vibrant mosaic of drama, spice, and unadulterated bliss. And as we dispersed into the dawning day, we carried the knowledge that within the embrace of music, friendship, and cultural exchange. The world becomes an extraordinary stage upon which the human spirit dances with unyielding fervor.

CHAPTER 5

A New Direction

The next morning arrived, accompanied by the harsh reality of a pounding headache and a queasy stomach—a clear consequence of the previous night's indulgence. As the persistent ring of the phone echoed through the room, I groaned and reluctantly reached for it. It was Ann once again, her voice filled with mischief.

"Hey, come over. Let's keep the party going," she suggested, her words laced with excitement.

I hesitated, feeling the weariness in my bones, and then mustered the courage to decline. "Thanks, Ann, but I think I'll pass today. My head is killing me from last night," I confessed, not willing to admit my hangover- induced weariness.

A glimmer of disappointment flickered in Ann's voice, but she quickly perked up and understood. "No worries, girl! Take care of yourself and have a good time at the mall. You deserve it!" she cheered, her words laden with understanding.

With Ann's well-wishes echoing in my mind, I made plans to spend the day at the mall with Jerry. We both shared a love for exploring sales and finding hidden gems amid the sea of discounted items. It was the perfect opportunity to indulge in some retail therapy and enjoy each other's company.

As we entered the bustling mall, our excitement grew. Jerry's eyes sparkled as he exclaimed, "Let's see what's on sale today! I have a feeling we're going to find some amazing deals."

I laughed, matching his enthusiasm. "Oh, you know I can never resist a good bargain. Lead the way, my shopping partner in crime!"

Hand in hand, we navigated through the vibrant stores, our laughter mingling with the chatter of fellow shoppers. With each discovery, our connection deepened, as we shared stories, offered opinions, and reveled in the joy of finding the perfect item at an irresistible price.

Amid the sea of shoppers, our rumbling stomachs reminded us of another important need—food. Jerry's eyes gleamed mischievously as he suggested, "Hey, I'm hungry. Want to get something to eat? There's a new restaurant here that I've been dying to try."

I nodded eagerly, my own hunger making its presence known. "Sounds like a plan! Lead the way, Jerry. I trust your impeccable taste in food as much as I trust your shopping skills."

We made our way to the restaurant, the aroma of tantalizing dishes wafting through the air. The cozy ambiance and friendly chatter created the perfect backdrop for what would become a memorable conversation.

Over a delicious meal, our voices intertwined in animated discussions. Suddenly, amid the clinking of cutlery, Jerry turned to me, his eyes filled with love and sincerity. My heart skipped a beat as he posed a question that caught me off guard.

"Do you want to get married?" he asked, his voice filled with a mix of nervousness and anticipation.

My eyes widened, and for a moment, time stood still. The euphoria of the weekend swirled around me, and in that enchanted moment, I couldn't help but feel the overwhelming love and joy that Jerry brought into my life. I responded with an enthusiastic "Yes!" that tumbled out of my mouth before I even had a chance to fully process the question.

A wave of emotions crashed over us as we basked in the realization that our lives were about to take an unexpected turn. The prospect of a future filled with love, commitment, and shared dreams filled me with a sense of euphoria. I looked into Jerry's eyes and felt an unshakable certainty that this was the right path for us.

As we continued our stroll through the mall hand in hand, I couldn't help but let my mind wander to our future wedding. Visions of vibrant colors, enchanting music, and mouthwatering cuisine danced in my imagination. I shared my thoughts with Jerry, a twinkle of excitement in my eyes.

"Can you imagine how beautiful it will be? I've always dreamt of a big wedding, surrounded by our loved ones, celebrating our love in grand style," I gushed, unable to contain my excitement.

Jerry's smile grew wider, mirroring my enthusiasm. "I want nothing more than to make your dreams come true. Let's plan an epic celebration—a testament to the love and happiness we've found together."

As we strolled hand in hand, admiring the displays and sharing dreams of our future, I couldn't help but reflect on the challenges and mistakes I had made in previous relationships. The end of my previous marriage had been a tumultuous period, and at times, I had sought solace in excessive drinking. I hardly ever drank while I was married. I was not a party girl. I used to look down on someone being drunk, and now I am doing me not caring about anything anymore. But finding Jerry had become a turning point, a beacon of light that guided me toward a happier, more fulfilling life.

Through our journey together, I had come to appreciate the importance of balance and nurturing relationships. The Labor Day weekend had served as a powerful reminder of the value of meaningful connections, both romantic and platonic. It had become a time of self-reflection and growth, setting the stage for a brighter future.

As the day drew to a close, we found solace in the knowledge that life's twists and turns had led us to each other—a partner who brought laughter, love, and a renewed sense of purpose. The weekend had been a transformative experience, reminding us to savor each moment and cherish the relationships that make life truly meaningful.

Looking back, I couldn't ignore the lessons I had learned along the way. Sometimes, we make decisions without fully thinking them through, especially when we're young and feeling invincible.

The mistakes of my past had shaped me, and the aftermath of my divorce had led me down a path of self-discovery. I had shed my judgmental views and realized the importance of living authentically, embracing who I truly was.

As I gazed into Jerry's eyes, filled with love and acceptance, I knew that I had found a partner who saw me for who I was, flaws and all. Together, we would embark on this new chapter unafraid of the challenges that lay ahead and fueled by the love and connection we shared.

CHAPTER 6

Reality of Prioritizing

As the years passed, I found myself at a crossroads, realizing that my priorities had evolved and shifted. Once, my main focus had been on work, paying bills, and ensuring my daughter's well-being. I was content with that, but deep down, I yearned for more in life. I had dreams of advancing in my career and even pursued higher education by enrolling in college.

However, the reality of balancing my responsibilities became overwhelming. Juggling classes while managing my daughter's school schedule proved to be a Herculean task. The long and arduous commute to work, battling the relentless city traffic every day, added to the mounting challenges. Eventually, I had to make a difficult decision and drop out of college, acknowledging that the timing wasn't right for me.

When my daughter graduated from high school, I toyed with the idea of giving education another try. But life had its own plans for me. I met an incredible man, my amazing boyfriend, and my attention shifted toward nurturing our blossoming relationship. It was a delightful coincidence when my daughter and I ended up in the same English class. We hadn't planned it, but there we were, sitting together and enjoying the learning experience as a duo.

In that class, we were given an assignment to write a first-person essay about someone special in our lives. I chose to write about my grandfather, a man who had played a profound role in saving my life.

When the professor asked us to exchange papers and have someone else read our work, I handed mine to my daughter. As she read my essay, she was taken aback. I had shared a deeply personal incident that she hadn't known about, and the revelation touched us both on a profound level.

It was during this exchange that my daughter expressed her desire for me to share more about my childhood in Trinidad. She wanted to know about my experiences, the adventures, and the friendships that shaped my early years. I happily obliged, diving into a treasure trove of memories. We laughed, we reminisced, and we cherished the simplicity and joy that defined that chapter of my life.

These heartfelt conversations with my daughter made me realize the importance of sharing our experiences and connecting through our stories. It became a reminder to treasure the past, to honor the moments that have shaped us, and to instill a sense of wonder and playfulness in our lives. As I embarked on this new chapter with Jerry, my boyfriend, I carried with me the invaluable lessons from the past, valuing the journey and the connections forged along the way.

Life had thrown unexpected curveballs, demanding that certain dreams be put on hold. But in the midst of it all, I discovered the beauty of living in the present moment, cherishing the people who brought joy into my life, and embracing the stories that make us who we are. My priorities had shifted, and I had learned to find happiness in the simplest of moments, celebrating love, laughter, and the genuine connections that make life truly meaningful.

With renewed determination, I embarked on this journey with Jerry, savoring each day and allowing the spicy flavors of life to add an extra kick to our experiences. Together, we embraced the unknown, appreciating the beauty of the present and weaving our stories into a tapestry of shared adventures. As I looked back on the path I had traveled, I was grateful for the detours and redirections that had led me to where I stood now—ready to embrace the future with open arms and a heart full of love.

CHAPTER 7

A Memorable Labor Day Weekend

After bidding Jerry farewell, I stepped out of the car and made my way to my front door. Physically and emotionally invigorated from the day's events, I couldn't help but feel a sense of fulfillment. Eager to wash away the remnants of the day, I indulged in a refreshing shower and carefully selected an outfit, wanting to look my best for the evening ahead.

As I arrived at my friend's house, the sound of laughter and music greeted me. The party was already in full swing, with tequila shots being passed around. Knowing my limits, I opted for vodka instead, wanting to maintain control and enjoy the evening without any regrets. My friend raised an eyebrow, noticing my drink choice.

"You do you," she said with a laugh. "We have plenty of tequila, but I respect your choice. Let's have a great time together."

And so we danced and laughed the night away, surrounded by the pulsating rhythms that filled the air. As the hours passed, more friends joined the gathering, and we ordered food to satisfy our hunger. The night was alive with joy and camaraderie, creating an electric atmosphere that seemed to suspend time.

Amid the revelry, I turned to my friend with a mischievous grin. "Hey, tomorrow is Monday. I don't want to drink too much. I need to be fresh for work on Tuesday."

My friends exchanged mischievous glances, instantly captivated by the idea. "Let's have a cookout on Monday!" they exclaimed, their enthusiasm infectious. Without hesitation, they entrusted me with organizing the event.

Determined to make it an unforgettable day, I swung into action. On Monday, we set off to the grocery store, stocking up on burgers, hotdogs, chickens, and all the fixings. The anticipation grew as we gathered our supplies and made our way to the river, our chosen spot for the day's festivities. It was the perfect setting to enjoy the outdoors and create lasting memories.

As we set up the grill, the tantalizing aroma of sizzling meat filled the air, blending with the sounds of laughter and splashing water. The river became our playground, offering moments of both serenity and exhilaration. We feasted on delicious food, taking breaks to swim, play games, and revel in the simple pleasures of the day.

With each passing hour, the bonds of friendship grew stronger. We shared stories, shared laughter, and embraced the freedom of the holiday. The sun shone brightly overhead, casting a warm glow upon our gathering. It felt as if time stood still, allowing us to fully immerse ourselves in the beauty of the moment.

As the sun began to set, painting the sky with vibrant hues, we gathered our belongings and bid farewell to the river. Contentment filled our hearts, surpassing any exhaustion that tugged at our bodies. The memories we had created would forever be etched in our minds, a testament to the power of friendship and the joy of shared experiences.

As I settled into bed that night, thoughts of the weekend's adventures swirled in my mind. It had been a Labor Day weekend unlike any other, a time of laughter, love, and personal growth. I couldn't help but acknowledge the invaluable lessons learned and the deep sense of appreciation I had gained for the present moment.

Life had a way of surprising us, leading us down uncharted paths and teaching us valuable lessons along the way. This memorable weekend served as a reminder to seize opportunities, nurture relationships, and embrace the simple joys that life offers. It was a celebration of the bonds that hold us together, a testament to the power of laughter, love, and cherished moments.

With a contented smile on my face, I closed my eyes, ready to rest and rejuvenate. Gratitude filled my heart as I drifted off to sleep, eagerly anticipating the new adventures and experiences that awaited me in the days to come.

PART 2

The Battle Begins

CHAPTER 8

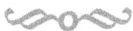

Back to Reality

Tuesday morning arrived, and with it came the return to work. As I groggily made my way to the kitchen, in desperate need of a cup of coffee, I was met with the familiar faces of my coworkers. They greeted me with warm smiles, genuine interest shining in their eyes as they inquired about my holiday weekend.

"It was amazing," I replied, a hint of excitement still lingering in my voice. "We had the most incredible time. The parties were wild, and we even ventured to the river for a day of fun. It was an absolute blast. And now, we're gearing up for the upcoming holidays—Thanksgiving and Christmas."

My coworkers chuckled and shared their own holiday experiences, each one bringing a mix of laughter and sighs. As we exchanged stories, a common theme emerged—a blend of joy and frustration, love, and exasperation.

"Oh, I know exactly what you mean," one coworker chimed in, a mischievous glint in her eyes. "I went out to lunch with my daughter, and she's already started making her extensive Christmas gift requests. It's unbelievable how their minds are always fixated on what else we can buy for them."

Mary, another coworker, let out a weary sigh. "Tell me about it. This new generation seems to be solely focused on themselves. They don't even consider if we can afford it or not. My daughter wants a MacBook, and on top of that, she has an endless list of other things she desires, right down to the smallest stocking stuffers. It's like they're so spoiled."

I nodded in agreement, understanding the struggle of balancing love and boundaries. "I completely understand," I replied. "My daughter has her own list too. It's important to set limits, but it's hard to resist their desires when we see that look of excitement in their eyes. Love makes it difficult to say no."

As our conversation delved deeper into the complexities of parenthood, the ringing of the phone abruptly interrupted our discussion. I hastily answered, slightly annoyed at the early hour. It was the breast center on the other end of the line, and my heart skipped a beat as they mentioned that my mammogram results were unclear and needed to be redone.

Confusion and concern washed over me like a tidal wave. I shared the unsettling news with Mary, her reassuring voice attempting to allay my fears. She explained that sometimes these things happen, that unclear results don't necessarily indicate a problem. Still, the worry lingered, clinging to my thoughts like a persistent shadow.

With a heavy heart, I made the necessary arrangements to go for the follow- up appointment during my lunch break. The weight of the impending appointment hung over me, an unwelcome companion that cast a pall over my day. The mundane tasks of work suddenly felt trivial, overshadowed by the uncertainty that loomed on the horizon.

In the midst of office chatter and the steady hum of productivity, my mind couldn't help but wander to the impending appointment. Questions swirled in my thoughts—What if the results were more than just unclear? What if there was something to be concerned about? The fear gnawed at me, threatening to consume my every waking moment.

But amid the anxiety, a glimmer of hope flickered. Mary's reassurance echoed in my mind, a beacon of possibility in the darkness. I held onto the belief that everything would turn out fine, that this was merely a bump in the road. With a deep breath, I returned to my work, determined to push through the day, all the while counting down the minutes until my lunch break—a moment that would bring either relief or a new set of challenges to face.

CHAPTER 9

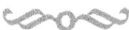

A Troubling Discovery

During my lunch break, I mustered up the courage to visit the medical center for the follow-up appointment. The technician informed me that we would be conducting an ultrasound this time, as the mammogram had not provided clear results. Curiosity and apprehension swirled within me, and I couldn't help but ask the technician why this happens at times.

With a kind and empathetic tone, the technician explained that mammograms may not always capture a clear image due to various factors, such as dense breast tissue or positioning during the procedure. These factors can make it challenging to obtain a definitive diagnosis. In such cases, additional tests, such as an ultrasound, are necessary to provide a more detailed view of the area in question. I nodded, trying to absorb the information, but a sense of unease lingered deep within me.

As the ultrasound began, it seemed to take longer than usual, and the technician's demeanor grew increasingly serious. An unspoken tension hung in the air, and I couldn't help but notice the worried glances exchanged between the technician and the doctor, intensifying my growing sense of unease. The room felt suffocating, and my heart raced with anticipation.

Finally, the door opened, and the doctor entered the room, her face bearing a grave expression.

She reviewed the ultrasound scans, her eyes carefully examining each image. The silence in the room was deafening, and my anxiety reached its peak. I held my breath, waiting for the doctor's verdict.

Time seemed to stretch on indefinitely before the doctor finally broke the silence, her voice filled with a mixture of concern and urgency. "A biopsy is required as soon as possible," she said, her words weighing heavily in the air. "The scans have revealed concerning areas that cannot be ignored."

Fear gripped me like a vice, and tears welled up in my eyes as the weight of the situation settled upon me. The room seemed to spin as a wave of panic surged through my body. Questions flooded my mind, and I struggled to comprehend the harsh reality of what I was facing. The thought of undergoing a similar experience to the patients I had treated as a trauma coodinator filled me with an overwhelming sense of dread.

In my profession, I had witnessed firsthand the challenges and hardships faced by patients battling various medical conditions. I had seen their strength, but I also knew the toll it took on them physically, mentally, and emotionally. Now, the possibility of going through that same ordeal myself was both daunting and terrifying.

With each passing day, the weight of anticipation grew heavier, and my mind became consumed with worry. The days felt like an eternity as I waited for the biopsy appointment, my thoughts swirling in a never-ending loop of fear and uncertainty. I longed for answers, desperate to know what lay ahead. Sleep became elusive, as my mind raced with countless scenarios and the what-ifs that plagued my thoughts. The nights were filled with restless tossing and turning. My dreams haunted by shadows of anxiety. The days, on the other hand, were a haze of numbness as I tried to navigate through the routine while grappling with the impending results.

The support of my loved ones became my lifeline during this challenging time. They offered words of comfort, a shoulder to lean on, and a listening ear for my fears and worries. Their presence reminded me that I was not alone in this battle, that there were people who cared deeply for me and would stand by my side no matter what.

As the day of the biopsy drew near, a mixture of emotions swirled within me—fear, hope, and a fierce determination to face whatever lay ahead. I held onto a glimmer of hope, clinging to the belief that no matter the outcome, I would find the strength and resilience to navigate this uncertain path.

The journey I found myself on was one of introspection, self-discovery, and resilience. I learned to cherish each moment, to find solace in the present, and to lean on the unwavering support of my loved ones. Life had a way of humbling us, reminding us of our own vulnerability, and teaching us to find strength in the face of adversity.

As I awaited biopsy, I held onto the notion that life was a tapestry woven with threads of both joy and sorrow. The road ahead was uncertain, but within the depths of uncertainty, I found a newfound appreciation for the preciousness of every breath, every heartbeat, and every moment of connection.

CHAPTER 10

The Road to Recovery

As the scheduled biopsy date approached, I found myself caught in the clutches of an all-consuming whirlwind of nervousness and anxiety. The mere thought of the impending procedure sent shivers down my spine, and each passing day seemed to magnify the weight of uncertainty that hung over me like a dark cloud. The day finally arrived, and I mustered all the strength I could summon to step into the sterile environment of the medical facility, my heart pounding with trepidation.

To my surprise, the doctor assigned to perform the biopsy not only exhibited exceptional medical expertise but also possessed a unique gift for comforting the weary souls of her patients. With her soothing words and empathetic demeanor, she managed to create a fleeting oasis of calm amid the turbulent storm of emotions swirling within me. It was as if she possessed an innate ability to sense the fears that plagued my mind and had made it her mission to alleviate them, if only for a brief moment.

As the morning unfolded, each biopsy seemed to serve as a stark reminder of the fragility of life. The sharp prick of the needle sent waves of discomfort coursing through my body, a physical manifestation of the emotional turmoil that had taken hold of me. The doctor, recognizing the toll it was taking on my spirit, looked at me with a compassionate gaze and uttered the words that provided a glimmer of relief: "You've been through enough for today. Return home and allow yourself the time and space to heal."

Physically and emotionally drained, I left the medical facility, my mind in a haze of exhaustion and anticipation. The waiting game had begun, and it felt as though time had transformed into a torturous adversary, taunting me with its sluggish pace. Each passing day felt like a lifetime, and the uncertainty gnawed at my spirit, threatening to unravel the fragile threads of hope I clung to.

In the midst of this prolonged limbo, I turned to my loved ones for solace.

Their unwavering support became a lifeline, anchoring me to reality as I battled against the demons of fear and doubt that threatened to engulf me. Their comforting presence and words of encouragement served as beacons of light amid the darkness, reminding me that I was not alone in this journey.

But the path to recovery was far from straightforward. It demanded unwavering resilience and an unwavering commitment to self-care. I sought solace in the simple pleasures of life, indulging in moments of respite that provided temporary reprieve from the weight of uncertainty. I poured my heart into activities that nurtured my soul, finding solace in creative pursuits, music, and the beauty of nature.

As the days turned into weeks, the anticipation reached a crescendo, the tension in the air nearly suffocating. The fear of what the results might reveal loomed over me, threatening to overshadow the flickering flame of hope that still burned within. But through it all, I clung to the belief that strength emerges from the depths of adversity, and I refused to surrender to the despair that whispered in the darkest corners of my mind.

The road to recovery was not a smooth one, marked by detours and unforeseen obstacles. But I vowed to forge ahead, armed with the unyielding determination to emerge from this chapter of my life stronger and more resilient than ever. I embraced each passing day as a test of my fortitude, holding onto the unwavering conviction that I was capable of conquering any challenge that dared to cross my path.

And so I trudged forward, my spirit unyielding, fueled by the fire of hope that refused to be extinguished. The road was treacherous, but within the depths of uncertainty, I discovered the boundless capacity of the human spirit to endure and overcome. With every breath, I drew closer to the revelation that awaited me, prepared to face whatever lay beyond the realm of uncertainty, armed with the knowledge that I had the strength to weather the storm and emerge on the other side, a testament to the indomitable power of the human spirit.

CHAPTER 11

The Unexpected News

Friday arrived, its mundane facade quickly shattered by the jarring ring of the phone. As the day unfolded, trembling hands reached out to answer the call, unknowingly stepping into the path of an emotional hurricane, my world was shattered by a phone call. The voice on the other end delivered the devastating news that would forever alter the course of my life—I had breast cancer, and it was an aggressive form of the disease, formidable adversary. Time seemed to slow to a crawl as the weight of those words sank deep into the recesses of my soul. I was left grappling with a flood of emotions— agony, pain, and doubt surged through my veins, threatening to consume me entirely.

In the days that followed, I found myself wandering through a disorienting haze of shock and disbelief. The ground beneath my feet felt unsteady, and the world around me appeared distorted and unfamiliar. The reality of my diagnosis seemed like a cruel twist of fate, an unwelcome intruder in the carefully constructed tapestry of my existence. I couldn't comprehend the reality of the situation. The mere thought of sharing this life-altering news with my loved ones filled me with immense fear. How would they react? How could I bear to witness their pain and anguish? The uncertainty of the future loomed over me like a dark cloud, threatening to engulf my hopes and dreams.

I sought solace in the solitude of my thoughts, grappling with the overwhelming uncertainty that loomed ominously over my future.

It felt as though I had been thrust into an alternate reality, one filled with medical jargon, treatment plans, and a constant undercurrent of fear. The unknown stretched out before me like an endless labyrinth, taunting me with its elusive promises and hidden perils.

With a heavy heart and great trepidation, slowly I mustered the courage to confide in my daughter, bracing myself for the emotional avalanche that would follow. Tears streamed down her face as the weight of the news settled upon her young shoulders. The pain we shared in that moment was indescribable, our intertwined hearts pulsating with a mixture of sorrow and determination. Together, we navigated the tumultuous waves of emotion, seeking solace in each other's arms and drawing strength from our unbreakable bond.

Weeks turned into months, and I found myself trapped in a state of oscillating doubt and denial. The looming specter of surgery, an invasive journey into the depths of my being, haunted my every waking thought. The prospect of losing a part of my body felt unbearable, an irrevocable loss that threatened to unravel the very fabric of my identity. Fear and uncertainty gnawed at my spirit, casting shadows of doubt over my ability to overcome this insidious foe.

In the midst of my despair, a familiar face emerged from the periphery of my professional world—a breast surgeon with whom I had crossed paths. Sensing my anguish, they extended a compassionate hand, their words a balm for my wounded soul. In lengthy conversations, they helped me confront my fears, unraveling the tangled threads of doubt that had ensnared me. They gently guided me toward a deeper understanding of the importance of taking decisive action. Reluctantly, I came to realize that surgery was not merely a harrowing ordeal; it was a vital step toward reclaiming my health, my future, and my very essence.

Still, my internal struggle persisted. Concentrating on my job became an arduous task, as grief clouded my thoughts, rendering my once-focused mind aimless and unfocused. Doubts and fears waged war within me, enticing me to cancel the surgery, to retreat from the painful reality that awaited. Yet deep within the recesses of my being, I knew that avoiding the situation would only prolong the inevitable.

Cancer was not an adversary to be wished away; it demanded immediate attention and action.

The days leading up to the surgery were fraught with an indescribable blend of anxiety and uncertainty. Doubts gnawed at me incessantly; their insidious whispers attempting to undermine my resolve. But within the depths of my being, a flicker of strength ignited, propelling me forward. I mustered the courage to face the unknown, to confront the fear head-on. The surgery loomed on the horizon like an imposing mountain, an inevitable confrontation that I had no choice but to endure. The thought of parting with a piece of my body felt like an insurmountable loss, but I clung to the hope that this step would ultimately save my life.

In the midst of this harrowing journey, I sought solace in the unwavering support of my loved ones. Their presence served as a sanctuary in a storm- ridden landscape, holding me up when my spirit faltered and providing a glimmer of light amid the darkest of nights. Together, we prepared ourselves for the impending surgery, recognizing the necessity of this difficult path toward healing and survival.

As I braced myself for what lay ahead, I knew that courage would be my guiding force. I steeled myself for the unknown, ready to face the challenges head-on. Breast cancer had thrust me into an unexpected battle—one that I never asked for nor anticipated—but I was determined to emerge from it stronger, armed with an unwavering resilience and an unyielding belief in the power of the human spirit to overcome even the most formidable of adversaries. It was through the crucible of this experience that I would forge a new understanding of strength, hope, and the extraordinary capacity of the human soul to transcend the limits imposed upon it.

And so I embarked on this arduous journey with an unwavering spirit, fortified by the love and support of those who held me up when my own strength faltered. Each step forward was a testament to the indomitable power of the human spirit, a testament to the resilience that resides within us all. In the face of uncertainty, I clung to the belief that healing and triumph were possible, that this chapter of my life would not define me, but rather refine me into an even stronger version of myself.

CHAPTER 12

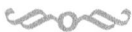

Surgery and Struggles

October 30, 2018, remains etched in my memory as a significant day in my journey—the day of my surgery. With a mixture of emotions and a sense of trepidation, I entered the hospital, mentally preparing myself for the challenges that lay ahead. The surgery itself was deemed a success, but the pain that followed served as a constant reminder of the battle I was fighting.

I spent a restless night in the hospital, surrounded by the comforting presence of my family and a few close friends. Their unwavering support and love provided a glimmer of solace amid the physical and emotional turmoil I was experiencing. Their presence reminded me that I was not alone in this journey and that together we could face whatever came our way. Their support became an anchor, grounding me in moments of uncertainty and providing strength when I needed it most.

On Halloween day, I was discharged from the hospital and returned home, stepping into a new reality marked by recovery and resilience. The road ahead was not easy, but I was determined to embrace the challenges with a spirit of courage and perseverance. I knew that the path to healing would require patience, self-compassion, and the support of my loved ones.

The days and weeks that followed were filled with moments of both triumph and struggle. The pain persisted, and the physical limitations imposed by the surgery served as a constant reminder of the battle my body had endured. Yet, even in the face of adversity, I held onto the belief that each day was a step closer to regaining my health and reclaiming my life.

Throughout my recovery, I leaned on my support system, cherishing their presence and drawing strength from their love. Their unwavering encouragement and willingness to lend a helping hand allowed me to navigate the challenges of daily life as I slowly regained my strength. Together, we celebrated small victories and pushed through setbacks, understanding that healing was a gradual process.

As the days turned into weeks and weeks into months, I witnessed my body's resilience and its capacity to heal. The pain began to recede, and I regained a sense of normalcy, albeit a new normal that incorporated the experiences and lessons of my journey. The surgery had marked a turning point, signaling a chapter of recovery and renewal.

Looking back, I am grateful for the love, support, and care that surrounded me during those challenging days. The surgery was not just a physical procedure; it was a testament to the power of community, compassion, and the indomitable spirit within me. It served as a reminder that even in the face of adversity, we have the capacity to heal and emerge stronger than before.

The road to recovery was far from easy, but with each passing day, I found solace in the resilience and strength that resided within me. It was through the support of my loved ones and my own determination that I continued to move forward, one step at a time. The journey was marked by both physical and emotional healing, and I emerged with a renewed sense of gratitude and a deep appreciation for the preciousness of life.

As I reflect on that significant day in my journey, I am reminded of the power of resilience, love, and the human spirit. Though the challenges were great, I am grateful for the strength and support that carried me through. And as I continue to heal, I embrace each day as an opportunity for growth, gratitude, and the pursuit of a life lived fully and authentically.

In those early days, the road to healing proved to be arduous. The pain became a constant companion, and the wounds left by the surgery served as a visual reminder of the battle I had waged within my own body. It was a challenging time, but I knew that there were steps I could take to restore what had been lost.

During this period, I visited a plastic surgeon to explore options for reconstruction. The prospect of undergoing additional surgeries felt daunting, but I held onto the hope of reclaiming a sense of normalcy and rebuilding my self-confidence.

The process of reconstruction was not in the cards, and it tested my patience and resilience. There were multiple surgeries involved, each with its own recovery period. It required a significant investment of time, energy, and emotional strength. However, I remained determined to move forward and restore what had been altered by the impact of cancer.

While the process felt prolonged and sometimes overwhelming, I found solace in the guidance and expertise of the medical professionals who supported me. They provided reassurance and a sense of security, helping me navigate the journey of reconstruction with care and compassion.

Throughout this process, I clung to the hope of regaining a sense of normalcy and reclaiming my physical appearance. I understood that the physical restoration was not only about aesthetics but also about restoring my self-image and confidence. It was a step toward embracing the changes and scars as symbols of strength and resilience rather than reminders of the battle I had fought.

It took time, patience, and ongoing self-compassion to navigate the challenges of reconstruction; however, I was still too weak. There were setbacks along the way, both physical and emotional, but I persevered, knowing that the end result would be worth it.

As the surgeries progressed, I began to see the transformation take shape. Each step brought me closer to a renewed sense of wholeness, both physically and emotionally. The wounds slowly healed. It was a testament to the resilience of the human body and spirit.

Reclaiming a sense of normalcy was not just about physical restoration but also about reclaiming my inner strength and embracing the changes I had undergone. It was about acknowledging the scars as a part of my journey and finding beauty and power in their presence.

As I moved forward on the path of healing, I carried with me the lessons learned, the strength gained, and the hope that propelled me forward. The process of reconstruction was a tangible reminder of my ability to overcome challenges and rebuild my life in the face of adversity.

Though the road was arduous, the surgeries served as stepping stones toward reclaiming my sense of self and embracing life with renewed optimism. It was a journey that tested my patience and resilience, but ultimately, it allowed me to find solace, strength, and a renewed sense of normalcy in the face of the challenges I had faced.

The next step on my journey was the oncologist's office—a place that held both dread and hope. As I sat in the waiting room, my heart pounding, I braced myself for the news that awaited me. When the doctor delivered the diagnosis, it felt like a punch to the gut—stage one cancer, but an aggressive form that required aggressive treatment. Chemotherapy loomed before me, a daunting journey that would span over a year.

The news was a heavy blow, and I struggled to process the magnitude of what lay ahead. I had no previous experience with chemotherapy, and the thought of enduring its side effects filled me with apprehension and uncertainty. My cancer had been identified as aggressive, leaving no room for complacency. Radiation therapy was not deemed necessary, but the chemotherapy regimen was essential to combat the insidious nature of the disease.

I chose to undergo my chemotherapy treatments at John Hopkins Hospital, seeking the best care and expertise available. As I embarked on this daunting chapter, I confronted the reality of the long road ahead—a road paved with physical and emotional challenges, yet also one illuminated by the strength and resilience within me.

The treatments would be grueling, testing my endurance and demanding great sacrifices. Yet within the walls of the hospital, I found solace in the compassion of the medical team and the unwavering support of my loved ones. They became my pillars of strength, reminding me that I was not alone in this fight.

As the journey unfolded, I discovered an inner wellspring of resilience and determination. Chemotherapy became a testament to my courage, an opportunity to confront the adversity that life had thrust upon me. Each treatment served as a battle won, a step closer to reclaiming my health and embracing the future with renewed hope.

Though the road ahead seemed daunting, I refused to let fear consume me. Instead, I focused on the possibility of healing, of emerging from this trial with a newfound appreciation for life and a profound gratitude for the strength that lies within each of us. John Hopkins Hospital became more than a place of medical care—it became a sanctuary of hope and resilience, where warriors like me fought battles both seen and unseen.

And so, armed with determination and the unwavering support of my loved ones, I took my place in the ranks of those who battle cancer, ready to face the challenges head-on and emerge stronger, both physically and emotionally.

CHAPTER 13

The Depths of Depression

As the weeks turned into months, and the chemotherapy's aftermath continued to take its toll, I found myself navigating the tumultuous landscape of my emotions. The side effects weighed heavily on my daily life, leaving an indelible mark on my physical and mental well-being. Each day brought a new battle, and I grappled with the lingering effects that seemed to cast a shadow over my existence.

One of the most significant challenges I faced was the impact on my memory. Short-term memory loss became a constant companion, casting a fog over my thoughts and making it difficult to recall even the simplest of details. But amid this struggle, there were still moments of joy and laughter that managed to penetrate the haze. I found solace in finding humor in the forgetfulness, and my loved ones rallied around me, creating lighthearted reminders and inside jokes to help ease the frustration.

Fatigue enveloped me, an unyielding weariness that seemed to seep into every fiber of my being. It was a different kind of exhaustion, one that could not be alleviated by rest alone. But, even in the midst of this fatigue, I discovered pockets of energy that allowed me to engage in activities that brought me joy. Whether it was painting, listening to music, or simply spending time in nature, these moments became precious bursts of vitality that reminded me of the beauty that still existed in the world.

Depression cast its dark shadow over my spirit, enveloping me in a deep sense of sadness and hopelessness. But within the depths of despair, I began to find small sparks of hope. Through therapy and support groups, I connected with others who had experienced similar journeys, and their stories of resilience and recovery inspired me. Together, we found solace in sharing our struggles and triumphs, and in those moments, the weight on my shoulders felt a little lighter.

Panic attacks became an unwelcome companion, striking unexpectedly and leaving me breathless and paralyzed by fear. But I refused to let fear define me. I sought out meditation and breathing exercises that helped me regain control of my breath and calm my racing heart. Slowly but surely, I learned to recognize the signs of an impending panic attack and developed strategies to ground myself in the present moment.

Through it all, my family remained a steadfast source of support. Their love and understanding provided a lifeline, anchoring me to a sense of purpose and reminding me that I was not alone in this struggle. My daughter, in particular, stood by my side, offering unwavering love and compassion. Our bond grew even stronger, forged in the fires of adversity. We found joy in simple moments together, whether it was sharing a heartfelt conversation or indulging in a favorite treat.

Time marched on, and we find ourselves in the year 2023. While I have made progress in my healing journey, the side effects still linger. Depression, fatigue, panic attacks, and other medical conditions continue to be part of my daily existence. But amid the challenges, I have learned to find joy. I have embraced the small victories and celebrated every step forward, no matter how small.

Though the road has been arduous and the scars remain, I choose to embrace the progress I have made. I am grateful for the support system that has sustained me, and I find solace in the moments of clarity and joy that punctuate my days. While the journey is far from over, I am determined to navigate it with courage, seeking beauty amid the challenges and embracing the lessons learned along the way.

As I move forward, I hold onto hope—a beacon of light in the midst of darkness. I am reminded that healing is not linear, and that it encompasses both triumphs and setbacks. With each passing day, I strive to cultivate self- compassion, finding strength in my resilience and embracing the beauty of a life lived with purpose, no matter the obstacles that may arise. And in this ongoing journey, I am determined to add more joy, spice, and drama— savoring the moments of laughter, embracing new experiences, and finding excitement in the twists and turns of life.

PART 3

Embracing Life and Giving Back

CHAPTER 14

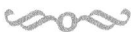

Lessons in Friendship and Gratitude

As I reflect on my journey of recovery, one of the most profound lessons I have learned is the true value of friendship and the power of gratitude. The experience of battling cancer exposed the stark reality that not everyone who claimed to be a friend would stand by my side during the darkest of times. It was a painful revelation, but one that ultimately led me to cherish the genuine connections in my life.

Before falling ill, I had lived a life filled with busyness and constant activity. Work and socializing had consumed my days, and I found myself spreading my time and energy thin. But when illness struck, it became clear who truly cared and who were mere acquaintances. I discovered that only a few friends and family members were there for me, offering unwavering support and love throughout the difficult journey.

These genuine connections became my lifeline, providing solace and strength when I needed it most. They were the ones who stood by me, offering a listening ear, a comforting presence, and genuine care. Their unwavering support became a beacon of light in the midst of darkness, reminding me that I was not alone.

In contrast, I witnessed the fading presence of those who had once occupied a prominent space in my life. As my battle with cancer intensified, they gradually faded into the background, their once-eager involvement replaced by distance and silence. It was a painful realization, but one that taught me a valuable lesson about the fickle nature of relationships.

Through this experience, I have learned to treasure the friends and family who remained by my side, offering love, support, and unwavering loyalty. I have come to understand the importance of cultivating deep connections, ones that stand the test of time and adversity. These individuals have become my true support system, and I now make a conscious effort to nurture these relationships with care and gratitude.

In the wake of my illness, I have adopted a practice of regularly checking in on those who have shown me kindness and support. I make it a priority to express my gratitude, whether through heartfelt conversations, small gestures, or acts of kindness. This deliberate effort to cultivate gratitude has deepened my connections, fostering a sense of reciprocity and love.

As I navigate life with the lingering side effects of my treatment, including depression, fatigue, and panic attacks, I am reminded of the fragility of health and the resilience of the human spirit. I continue to seek support from my loved ones and medical professionals, acknowledging that healing is an ongoing process.

Though my journey has been challenging, it has also brought forth profound growth and self-discovery. I have learned to appreciate the power of authentic connections, the importance of gratitude, and the resilience within me. As I move forward, I carry these lessons with me, cherishing the relationships that have sustained me and embracing life with a renewed sense of purpose and gratitude.

During this time, I prioritize open communication with my loved ones about my experiences and challenges. They offer me emotional support, understanding, and companionship as I navigate these lingering effects. Sharing my feelings and concerns with them helps alleviate the burden I may be carrying.

Additionally, I connect with medical professionals who specialize in supporting individuals with post-treatment side effects. They provide guidance, offer treatment options, and help me manage my physical and mental health. I don't hesitate to reach out to my healthcare team to discuss my symptoms and explore potential solutions.

I remember that healing is a multifaceted journey that requires patience and self-compassion. I allow myself to prioritize self-care and seek activities that bring me joy and relaxation. Engaging in activities like meditation, gentle exercise, creative pursuits, or spending time in nature helps alleviate my symptoms and promote overall well-being.

I explore therapeutic techniques, such as cognitive-behavioral therapy (CBT) or mindfulness-based practices, which provide me with tools and strategies to cope with negative thoughts, physical symptoms, and overwhelming emotions.

As I navigate life with these challenges, I remind myself that I am not alone. There are support groups, online communities, and organizations dedicated to providing resources and a sense of community for individuals facing similar experiences. Connecting with others who share my journey provides me with a valuable support network and an opportunity to exchange coping strategies and insights.

Finally, I embrace the understanding that healing is a personal and ongoing process. I am patient with myself, allowing for setbacks and celebrating small victories along the way. I trust in my own resilience and continue to seek the support and resources that contribute to my well-being.

Every day is an opportunity to nurture the bonds that have uplifted me, to show appreciation to those who have been there through thick and thin. I find joy in creating meaningful experiences with my loved ones, whether it's shared laughter, adventures, or simply being present in each other's lives.

I have come to understand that life's challenges can teach us valuable lessons and shape us into stronger individuals. I embrace the journey, cherishing the relationships that have withstood the test of time and adversity. And as I navigate the ups and downs that come my way, I do so with a heart full of gratitude, knowing that I am surrounded by love and support.

Friendship and gratitude have become guiding principles in my life, reminding me to cherish the bonds I have and to express my appreciation for the kindness and compassion that has been bestowed upon me.

Through the highs and lows, I continue to cultivate and nurture these connections, knowing that they are an invaluable source of strength, joy, and comfort.

As I move forward, I carry the lessons learned in my heart, forever grateful for the true friends who have stood by me and the power of gratitude that has illuminated my path. Each day is an opportunity to embrace life, to embrace the relationships that enrich my journey, and to live with a spirit of gratitude and love.

CHAPTER 15

Celebrating Life

Now I live my life differently. I spend time with family and friends and not party till morning light. I guess God did this to slow me down. Well, he did a good job.

I spend more time with my daughter than I ever have before. We have cultivated close bonds built on trust, love, and mutual understanding. Watching my daughter grow into a remarkable young woman fills me with pride and gratitude. Together, we navigate the ups and downs of life, supporting and loving one another unconditionally.

My daughter, with her boundless love and compassion, has stood by my side throughout my journey. Her presence brings me immeasurable joy, and her unwavering support reminds me of the beauty and strength of our bond. We share precious moments together, cherishing the laughter, love, and shared experiences that bring light to my days.

My daughter and Jerry have become my greatest joys and sources of inspiration. Their unwavering support anchors me during challenging times, and Jerry has become my rock.

And then there's Jerry, who has been a steadfast presence throughout it all. His unwavering support and love have been a constant source of strength for me. He stands by my side, offering a listening ear, a comforting presence, and an unwavering loyalty. His unwavering belief in me and his dedication to our relationship have been an anchor during the most challenging times.

Jerry's support is a reminder that I am not alone in my journey. His presence gives me courage and helps me navigate the ups and downs with resilience and determination. Together, we face the challenges head-on, finding solace and strength in each other.

In moments of darkness, when depression and fatigue threaten to overwhelm me, Jerry's unwavering support becomes a beacon of light. His love and encouragement lift me up, reminding me of the strength I possess within. With him by my side, I feel a sense of security and comfort that helps me face each day with renewed hope.

As I continue to navigate the lingering effects of my treatment, Jerry's presence and support are invaluable. He provides a sense of stability, understanding, and unwavering love that propels me forward on my healing journey. His belief in me fuels my determination to overcome the challenges I face.

I am grateful for the love and support of both my daughter and Jerry. They bring immense joy and inspiration into my life. With their love and presence, I find the strength to face each day with courage, resilience, and gratitude. Together, we navigate life's challenges, cherishing the moments of joy and growth that emerge along the way.

Through this journey, I have also learned to discern who truly stands by my side. It is a valuable lesson in understanding the depth of relationships and the significance of genuine support. I have let go of those who were merely present during the good times, realizing that it is the ones who stay through the storms that truly matter.

I always thought I had it all together, but little did I know I had nothing together. Every year since then, I have celebrated something called Celebration of Life. In the end, it's about this beautiful life God gave us. It's up to us to choose which road we take, and I choose life and enjoying the nature of life, God's creation.

Over time, I realized the importance of celebrating life's milestones. I started an annual tradition of Celebration of Life, commemorating the day I received my diagnosis. Surrounded by loved ones, including my incredible daughter and supportive partner, Jerry, we rejoice in the gift of life and the strength that carried me through my darkest days.

It is a time to gather with family and friends, expressing gratitude for their unwavering support and love. We celebrate the journey we have taken together, filled with love, resilience, and the power of genuine connections.

I have come to understand that life is a precious gift, and it is our responsibility to make the most of it. Gone are the days of partying until the early hours of the morning. Instead, I prioritize quality time spent with my loved ones, creating lasting memories and forging deeper connections.

God, in His infinite wisdom, guided me on this path for a reason. He slowed me down and shifted my priorities, allowing me to rediscover the beauty and blessings that surround me. I have learned to appreciate the simple joys of life, the wonders of nature, and the marvels of God's creation.

Reflecting on the journey, I now recognize that even the smallest moments have the power to transform lives. A simple act of kindness, a heartfelt conversation, or a shared laughter can bring light to the darkest of times. It was a mere $50.00 that saved my life.

As I continue to navigate life with its challenges and uncertainties, I am grateful for the perspective gained through adversity. I have emerged stronger, more resilient, and with a deep appreciation for the beauty that exists in the everyday.

Life is a tapestry of experiences, both triumphs and tribulations. It is up to us to choose how we navigate this journey. And for me, I choose life— embracing each day with gratitude, celebrating the connections that bring me joy, and finding solace in the unwavering love of my daughter and Jerry.

In the end, it was not the material possessions or the pursuit of worldly ambitions that mattered. It was the love, the relationships, and the celebration of life that truly made a difference. And with each passing year, as I mark the Celebration of Life, I am reminded of the preciousness of this existence and the profound impact it has had on my soul.

CHAPTER 16

The Gift of Giving

Inspired by my own journey, a newfound purpose emerged within me—to give back and make a difference in the lives of others. I recognized the significance of supporting those who were fighting their own battles against breast cancer, just as I had.

Driven by gratitude and a deep desire to make an impact, I made the decision to donate $50 each year to the cancer foundation that played a crucial role in saving my life. I understood that my donation might not be the largest, but I firmly believed that every act of giving, regardless of size, carries the potential to create a ripple effect of positivity.

For me, the act of donating was about more than just the monetary value. It was a symbol of my appreciation for the care and support I had received. It was a way to show solidarity with others who were facing similar challenges, to provide hope, and to remind them that they were not alone in their fight against breast cancer.

In giving, I found a sense of healing for myself as well. It allowed me to channel my own experiences and pain into something meaningful and uplifting. Through my donations, I aimed to inspire others to join in the cause to spread awareness about breast cancer, and to support those who were affected by it.

I knew that even a small contribution could make a difference. It could fund research, provide resources for patients, or support programs that offer emotional and practical assistance. Every dollar had the potential to contribute to advancements in treatment and care.

Moreover, my hope was that my act of giving would encourage others to get involved in their own ways. Whether it was through donations, volunteering, or raising awareness, I believed that together we could make a significant impact in the lives of individuals and families affected by breast cancer.

Through my annual donations, I aimed to create a legacy of compassion, gratitude, and support. I wanted to be part of a movement that brought about positive change and empowered others to take action. Breast cancer had profoundly impacted my life, and I was determined to use my experiences to make a difference in the lives of others.

In the end, my act of giving was not solely about the monetary contribution, but about the message it conveyed. It was a testament to the strength of the human spirit, and a reminder that even in the face of adversity, we can choose to come together and uplift one another. It was a way to express my gratitude, to honor the care I received, and to give back to a cause that had touched my life so deeply.

Beyond financial contributions, I recognized that my story and experiences could serve as a source of hope and inspiration for others facing similar challenges.

Sharing my story became a powerful way to raise awareness and foster a sense of community. By sharing my vulnerabilities, triumphs, and lessons learned, I aimed to provide comfort and reassurance to those who were navigating their own battles with breast cancer.

Offering words of encouragement became a vital part of my commitment to making a difference. I reached out to individuals I met through support groups, online communities, or social media, providing a listening ear and a compassionate voice. I understood firsthand the importance of having someone to turn to during difficult times, and I wanted to be that support for others.

In the near future, I see myself participating in fundraising events. It will allow me to contribute to important researches, patient support programs, and initiatives aimed at raising awareness. These events not only provided financial support but also created a sense of unity and camaraderie among participants, reminding everyone that they were part of a larger movement.

By giving my time and energy to various endeavors, it will feel like a deep sense of fulfillment and purpose. It is a way for me to actively engage with the breast cancer community, to extend a helping hand, and to create positive change. These acts of service became an integral part of my commitment to making a difference and leaving a lasting impact.

In giving my time, sharing my story, and offering support, I aimed to inspire others to join the cause, to raise awareness, and to support those affected by breast cancer. I understood that collectively, our efforts could create a ripple effect, reaching individuals and communities far beyond what I could achieve on my own.

Through these actions, I hoped to be a beacon of hope, resilience, and compassion. I wanted to show others that their stories mattered, that their voices were powerful, and that they were not alone in their journey. By giving of myself, I found fulfillment in knowing that I could make a positive impact in the lives of others.

In the end, giving my time and energy became a testament to the strength of the human spirit and the power of unity. It was an embodiment of my commitment to making a difference, one step at a time. Whether through contributing financially, sharing my story, or offering support, I strived to be a source of hope and inspiration, leaving a lasting legacy of compassion and resilience in the fight against breast cancer.

As the years passed, I witnessed the impact of my giving firsthand. I saw the smiles on the faces of patients receiving care, the hope kindled in their hearts, and the sense of community that was built through shared experiences. It was a reminder that our collective efforts, no matter how small, can bring about significant change and provide a glimmer of light in the midst of darkness.

The act of giving became a way for me to pay forward the love and support that had been bestowed upon me during my own battle with breast cancer. It allowed me to extend a helping hand, to offer comfort and guidance, and to remind others that they were not alone in their journey.

In the process of giving, I also discovered a sense of fulfillment and purpose that went beyond my personal struggles. It became a source of strength and resilience, as I saw firsthand the resilience and courage of those fighting breast cancer.

Through the gift of giving, I not only transformed the lives of others but also experienced my own transformation. It reaffirmed my belief in the power of compassion, the strength of community, and the importance of finding meaning even in the midst of adversity.

As I continued to navigate life, grateful for each day and the blessings it brought, I remained committed to my journey of giving. Whether through financial contributions, volunteering, or simply offering a listening ear, I knew that even the smallest acts of kindness could have a profound impact on someone's life.

Breast cancer had forever changed me, but it had also opened my eyes to the immense power of giving and the resilience of the human spirit. Through my annual donations and acts of service, I hoped to inspire others to embrace the gift of giving, to spread love and support, and to make a difference in the lives of those who needed it most.

And as I reflected on my own journey, I found solace in the knowledge that the greatest gift we can give is not just our resources but also our empathy, compassion, and unwavering support. In doing so, we create a world where no one fights alone, where hope thrives, and where the gift of giving becomes a catalyst for healing and transformation.

Epilogue

The Power of a $50 Bill

My journey was a rollercoaster ride, filled with ups and downs, moments of pain, and moments of joy. Through it all, I learned invaluable lessons about the strength of love, the importance of family, and the indomitable spirit of the human soul. But perhaps most significantly, my story became a testament to the transformative power of a simple $50 bill.

That seemingly insignificant piece of currency held the power to change the course of my life. It was that $50 bill that motivated me to schedule the wellness check that ultimately led to the early detection of breast cancer. In the face of uncertainty, that small act of seeking medical advice propelled me towards a new perspective on what truly matters.

I often wonder what would have happened if I had brushed aside the importance of that $50 bill. If I had chosen to ignore the nudge to prioritize my health. But I am forever grateful that I listened to that inner voice urging me to take action.

That $50 bill served as a reminder of the profound impact even the smallest choices can have. It taught me that sometimes, it's the seemingly insignificant decisions that shape the trajectory of our lives. It's the moments of courage and vulnerability that pave the way for transformative experiences.

As I reflect upon my journey, I am humbled by the power of that $50 bill. It wasn't just about the monetary value; it was about the message it carried— the message of taking care of oneself, of being proactive, and of valuing one's own well-being. That $50 bill symbolized the importance of self-care and self-advocacy, and it became a catalyst for change in my life.

Through my story, I hope to inspire others to recognize the power they hold within themselves. To understand that even the smallest choices can have profound consequences. I encourage everyone to listen to that inner voice, to prioritize their health, and to take action when it matters most.

Life is a fragile gift, and it's up to us to make the most of it. My journey taught me to appreciate the love and support of my family, the strength of my relationships, and the resilience of the human spirit. It reminded me that amid the chaos and uncertainty, there is always hope, and there is always an opportunity for growth and transformation.

So, as I move forward, I carry the lessons learned from my journey. I embrace the power of a $50 bill and the significance it holds in my life. I cherish the love and support of my family, the unwavering bond with my daughter, and the rock-solid presence of Jerry by my side.

And with a heart filled with gratitude, I face each new day, knowing that my story and the power of a simple $50 bill will continue to inspire others to prioritize their own well-being, to seek support and love, and to cherish the precious gift of life

Milton Keynes UK
Ingram Content Group UK Ltd.
UKHW031830010924
447661UK00001B/138